NLP For Beginners:

Neuro-Linguistic Programming Techniques Essential Guide to Treat and Overcome Depression, Cold, Allergies, Bad Habits, Illnesses and Disorders

By

Eva Delano

Table of Contents

Introduction 5

Chapter 1. NLP Basics 6

Chapter 2. Adjusting Negative Behaviors 8

Chapter 3. Creating Positive Behavior 14

Chapter 4. Positive Affirmation 16

Chapter 5. How to Improve Your Performance 21

Conclusion 26

Thank You Page 27

NLP For Beginners: Neuro-Linguistic Programming Techniques Essential Guide to Treat and Overcome Depression, Cold, Allergies, Bad Habits, Illnesses and Disorders

By Eva Delano

© Copyright 2015 Eva Delano

Reproduction or translation of any part of this work beyond that permitted by section 107 or 108 of the 1976 United States Copyright Act without permission of the copyright owner is unlawful. Requests for permission or further information should be addressed to the author.

This publication is designed to provide accurate and authoritative information in regard to the subject matter covered. This work is sold with the understanding that the publisher is not engaged in rendering legal, accounting, or other professional services. If legal advice or other expert assistance is required, the services of a competent professional person should be sought.

First Published, 2015

Printed in the United States of America

Introduction

In the following pages, we will explore some of the ways NLP can help each person live a better life. We will explore the fundamental steps required to make a change in one's life. We will also consider a few techniques within NLP to better understand how the process works and how it is relevant to self development. Finally, in the last pages, we will perform a simple NLP exercise together so that it becomes perfectly clear what NLP can do for you; or rather what NLP can help you to do for yourself.

This can be considered an introduction into the power, use, and application of NLP principles, but even this basic information will prove extremely powerful. Mental health, physical well being, successful personal development, and even learning and developing new skills and talents, can all be enhanced and achieved through practice of NLP. You are invited to learn more. Please continue on.

Chapter 1. NLP Basics

Neuro-Linguistic Programming is an integrated system used to identify areas in one's life which can be improved, and then taking a series of steps to realize those goals. It can be an extremely powerful system when applied by a knowledgeable practitioner, it can fundamentally alter the way one live, and it can be learned by anyone. The tools and steps entailed in successful NLP practice are the same for everyone, and they can be learned by anyone. Once mastered (and this can be accomplished in a fairly short time) these techniques can be applied to resolve issues with mental disorder, colds/allergies/flu, chronic medical conditions, psychosomatic disorders (hint: they're all psychosomatic) phobias, and even something as simple as shyness.

NLP goes beyond treating disorders however. This technique can be applied to your daily life, in order to maximize your potential to become your best self. NLP techniques can help you to become a better listener, better communicator, and more influential speaker. They can improve your physical wellness, vigor, and life energy. These techniques can even be applied in order to learn new skills and abilities. These outcomes are within the reach of every human, and all that is needed is training and practice in the techniques. Once the concept has been mastered, you can achieve whatever you truly set your mind to.

Originally developed as a psychotherapy technique, its developers Bandler and Grinder, quickly began to see the broader potential for such a powerful tool. After several adjustments to the overall practice, they began introducing individuals to the practices of NLP, not in a therapist-client relationship, but rather to empower individuals to help themselves. Their goal was that each individual would be able to live to their highest potential, and that each individual would have the means to guide themselves through a system of constant self development. Even though it all began in the 1970's, the fundamental principles still apply, as true now as they ever will be.

Chapter 2. Adjusting Negative Behaviors

Negative behaviors are not something any of us need to live with. These are any type of behavior that you are aware of, but yet feel powerless to change: phobias, shyness, bad habits (e.g. smoking), unhealthy eating practices, eating disorders, depression, anxiety, laziness, and even loneliness. These can all be adapted through application of NLP techniques, and you'd be amazed how quickly they can be overcome; sometimes success is realized in only a single session.

Your thoughts lead to your actions. Fortunately, you can control the way you think. Therefore, with careful attention to the way you think, you can manipulate what you think, and thereby affect the results of your thinking – namely your actions and experiences. In this section, we are discussing ways to adjust negative behavior; let's take a second to define *negative*.

A negative behavior is any action or result that has come about mindlessly. In one sense (though in no profound manner) a simple case of the hiccoughs might exemplify a negative behavior. My body is acting in a way that I do not value, which I did not ask it to do, and which is having an obvious effect on my overall existence. If the hiccoughs were intentional, and they were what I wanted to experience at that time, then they would not be negative (this is not a value judgment, merely assigning personal responsibility for the results of my thoughts). If the hiccoughs were unintentional, but had no noticeable impact on my life, then perhaps we could say that they are a neutral phenomenon (though later in our practice we would no longer accept that cop-out). Finally, if the hiccoughs were precisely what I had decided to experience at that time, they of course would not be negative, because mind-body integration is one of the fundamental goals of NLP (as well as a founding principle).

So we have identified a negative behavior that we'd like to adjust. Notice, we're not fighting the behavior itself, as behavior is merely the result of thought. Nor are we attempting to 'eliminate' the behavior. Our goal is simply to bring our behavior and experience closer in line with our goals and expectations. For example, let us set out to adjust our interactions with strangers.

We must honestly take stock in how we perceive an interaction with a stranger, and to do that, we must utilize our five senses, and our inherent natural language. Our five senses: sight, hearing, smell, taste, and touch are our chief means of interpreting our external world. We then tie those experiences together into a fabric of reality by using some type of internal language. Later in life, sometime around age 2 or so, we start to identify an external language with our internal language, and then we start speaking.

So, we process our negative behavior (meeting a stranger) through our five senses. What do I see when I look at someone I don't know. What do they sound like to me. Do my hands feel sweaty, my mouth dry or wet…do they smell strange? We put ourselves fully into the situation by using our senses and our natural language (the language we use to speak to ourselves in our own head). Now, when we think of our negative behavior, it is no longer an abstract idea, but rather a palpable sensory experience. At this point, when we feel "meet a stranger" we have identified the behavior which we will soon adjust.

Next we will identify our desired outcome. At first, this can be difficult for many people, as they often describe the desire as simply an absence of the unwanted…however if we once again use our senses to identify what that outcome would be, we realize that it cannot simply be an absence. So, we may choose to see the stranger as they are; they have hair, and a certain type of skin, and certain clothing, etc. They smell strange to you, because you have not met, so that's ok. Simply be aware of the strangeness of their smell. How does their voice sound? Familiar or unfamiliar? Maybe it reminds you of someone you know, or a celebrity. We construct a picture of how we will engage our five senses upon meeting a stranger, and what that will feel like. Once we know the desired feeling of our adjusted behavior, we have targeted a goal.

At this point, we have clearly defined, using our senses, both the behavior we want to adjust, and the goal we are targeting for the adjusted behavior. Without taking the time to carefully and explicitly define these two steps for yourself, the rest of your efforts will absolutely come to nothing. Without clear goals and objectives, there can be no clear result; often times there will be no result at all, save confusion, frustration, and a feeling of 'lostness'.

The next practice, and the final internalized step, is to project. Take a moment, clear your mind (as best you can) and project forward to the first time you experience the conditions of your negative behavior (meeting a stranger). The more thorough this projection is, the more powerful this session will be. If you are able to genuinely project, then you may adjust your behavior in a single session…in the beginning, when your ability to project is muddled, it may take some practice. But, employing the same sensory clarity you used to identify your behaviors, picture your conditions. Where are you, what does the stranger look like, sound like, smell like, etc. How does the air feel around you, are there any ambient environmental sounds. Now, at the same time, realize your sensory goals for this event. For this experiment, the goal was to simply assess the situation without judgment or upset. In your future projection, behave exactly as you wish to behave…and be sure to feel that action with your senses. By feeling yourself act in the way of your positive goal, you speak internally with the natural voice, and through that process you learn a new way of existing. Once your inner-self learns a new way of action, your behavior has been adjusted. There is no chance of 'forgetting', or 'relapse'. In fact, this new behavior will remain as natural to you as breathing until or unless you decide to adjust it further.

This technique can be applied to smoking, to getting sick around cold/flu season, to the bodies propendency to overact to external stimuli (allergies), to adjust depressive or self loathing thoughts, defeatism, over-eating...any condition in your life which you are able to describe to yourself on a deep sensory level, and for which you are able to describe a positive behavioral goal, can be carried through this process. The more you practice, the better you get. Start small, and work your way up to the big stuff.

Chapter 3. Creating Positive Behavior

Creating positive behavior is even easier than adjusting negative behaviors. As you probably guessed, it begins with defining a goal. In this case, let's say we want to spend one hour each day in low exertion exercise (walking, push-up/sit-up, swimming, etc). The mistake many people make, and the one that always leads to failure, is to justify the decision- "it'll be good for my health, it will help me manage my stress, i will feel better about myself". While these justifications seem true, seem honorable, and seem like the perfect medicine to motivate you toward your goal, in the end they are still justifications. We are not interested, in NLP, in justifying decisions. We simply define goals and then construct or adjust the behaviors in order to experience the desired results. Perhaps your goal setting process might include the reasons for deciding to exercise one hour each day. Setting meaningful and relevant goals is absolutely necessary for a sense of well being especially early in your process of NLP. Eventually, you will feel confident to set any goal you choose. Goal setting, like every other step in this system, is a skill that must be developed and honed over time, through diligent and mindful practice.

By applying your wants and needs to the goal setting process, you can arrive at a meaningful and attainable goal. However, once you set your goal, there needs be no further consideration of 'why'. Just as with adjusting a negative behavior, we need to use our five senses to process and understand our goal. How do I feel when I make the decision to go exercise. What am I wearing. Which activity have I just completed prior to making my decision (was I watching TV, finishing a meal, getting home from work) How does it feel to be exercising (maybe I'm sweating, my lungs ache a bit, I smell my own body). The more complete your sensory vision of the desired goal, the faster you will program yourself to achieve that result.

Developing positive behaviors, in conjunction with adjusting negative behaviors, is the way to realize your goals in life. Your thoughts lead to actions, your actions breed results. The circumstances of your life are the direct consequent of your thoughts and beliefs.

Chapter 4. Positive Affirmation

This is a concept that has been abused, misused, misrepresented, and much maligned over the last half-century. Somehow it became synonymous with 'wishful thinking' or 'positive thought manifestation'. Somehow, people began to believe that by simply holding a thought in their head, or repeating it out loud, that it would come true. Of course, this is nonsense. I can sit around and wish for an apple all day, but chances are pretty good it's not going to do anything to get me an apple. This is because we are skipping some important steps in the process of achieving our goals...namely incorporating our senses, and letting our actions drive our results.

Let's take a look at positive affirmation through a simple and practical example of its use. Let's say it's flu season where you live, and you really don't enjoy having the flu. Now, it's silly to believe that simply by 'hoping' you don't get the flu (everyone *hopes* they don't get it) or by deciding you don't want the flu (few people *want* it) that you will remain healthy that season. Rather, let's apply the same principles, the true principles of NLP, to set, identify, and achieve our goal.

To begin with, let's consider our goal. Our goal cannot be 'to not get the flu' because that is simply an absence. You can't hope to achieve 'not flu' because 'not flu' doesn't exists. Rather, you will to set a tangible goal, a goal you can actually achieve. Maybe your goal is to maintain health throughout this flu season (seems silly to limit health only to a certain season…but one step at a time). So already, we've made a series of powerful revelations regarding our goals. I am not concerned with flu or not-flu, but rather my goal orients on health; specifically my goal is to maintain health. Second, I realize that I don't simply want to maintain health for the next 6 weeks during flu-season, but rather that i wish to maintain health all the time (this becomes part of a system of ongoing self development, but that's a little more advanced practice). So, in the simplest sense, my goal has become, 'I am deciding to remain at my current health level –now'.

To make this a meaningful goal, one must experience fully their current health level (or if you wish to become healthier, then you must experience the level of health you desire to attain). Using your senses, experience fully how it feels to be you, to be healthy. My vision is clear and acute, I breathe slowly, calmly, and deeply. I feel the cool air flow through my nose and into my lungs. My skin feels cool and alive, not dry or clammy, or hot. My head feels clear, my hearing is crisp. Spend time feeling yourself and understanding the state of wellbeing that you wish to maintain. Again, the deeper your understanding of what 'health' means to you at this time, the more powerful your ability to maintain health at that level. And of course, you can always go back later and decide to be even healthier.

Now that you have a total mind-body understanding of what you've decided 'health' is, and you understand that your goal is to maintain health at this level, then it comes time to assign your affirmation to this positive state. The wording of this statement is of particular importance, because it will reflect the results you achieve.

Consider the following: "I want to remain healthy" If this is your affirmation, then what you'll achieve is the desire to be healthy. That is what you will actually actualize. You will find yourself wishing that you could be in the state of health that defined for yourself in the earlier exercise of establishing your goal. Whatever your affirmation, it is the only thing you are likely to achieve. Likewise, consider this: "I will remain healthy" Again, this seems fine, however it makes no sense. You will remain healthy? When will that happen? Or even this mistaken mantra of fear "I'm not getting sick, I'm not getting sick…" That's nonsense too…it fails to preclude the idea that you are already sick.

Earlier we defined what 'healthy' means to us by exploring the state of health fully with our senses. Now we will couple that understanding to a functional affirmation in order to use our understanding to power our behavior, and thus ensure desired results: "I am remaining in a healthy state" -or- "I am not moving from my state of health". These allow your body a reference point. You have defined what 'health' is. You have decided to stay that way for now. In doing so, any divergence from that state, for better or worse, runs counter to your decision. Bacteria, viruses, allergens, toxins, etc may pass through your body (we cannot avoid exposure to these things) but they will not have any impact on your state of health as you defined it. That is why it is so important to take the time to create meaningful understanding of your goals through application of the senses. If to you, 'health' is merely a normal temperature, then you leave room for all types of symptoms to affect you. If, however you take the time to get down to the minutiae of what health means to you, then you will maintain your health in every manner that is important to you.

Likewise, when people wake up in the morning and say to themselves, today I will be successful, or today I will lose weight, or today I will get a job…they are wasting their time until they stop to examine what that means, learn to understand what achieving that goal feels like through their senses, and construct a meaningful affirmation which actually describes the state of being in which the decide to exist. It isn't magic, it's hard introspective declarative work that must be carried out by a precise and present mind.

Chapter 5. How to Improve Your Performance

Think of an athlete; they practice their sport, but they also undergo all manner of training that aids them in performing the application of the sport itself. The same is true of a musician, and artist, a chef…anyone who employs a practiced skill also spends a great deal of time in enhancing the supportive characteristics of that skill. Now, NLP is a powerful skill which can be used, not to shoot a 3-pointer, or bake a souffle, but rather to live and be the life and person that you decide to live and be. It is a way to apply your skills of experience and employ the energy of your mind/internal self, to condition behavior, in order to realize results. Just like any other skill, the practitioner of NLP will benefit greatly by enhancing the cursory skills necessary to fully employ their inherent ability.

Focus: Training yourself to focus will help tremendously in your sensory-definition phases. It is necessary that the practitioner of NLP be able to delve into their sensory experience in order, not only to set goals, but also to practice them through future-projection exercises, as well as employ those actions under real life circumstances (until it becomes learned behavior) For this, highly developed focus makes a tremendous difference.

One simple exercise is to participate in sensory-consciousness. This is simple and fun, and goes a great way to inform you of your own senses. All you need to do is be aware of yourself, as you become aware of your surroundings. Breath in, and feel your breath. Is is hot, warm , cooling? Can you detect any odor? Flowers, car exhaust, a distant rain? Do not assign qualities to the things you experience, they are neither good nor bad...simply it is good and true that you are experiencing them. Look around you; what do you see -- *how do you see?* What is it like to be able to see and what happens when you close your eyes. Play the same game with hearing, with touch, with taste. Play it every day. No one needs to know. You can do it at work, at home, in the car or a hospital bed, or when you lay down to sleep. Likely, you will find it relaxing and calming at first. At some point you may find it thrilling and invigorating to finally wake-up to your own senses. This is the energy you will utilize later in defining your goals and behaviors. Go on...try it now.

Be Aware of Self: Another similar exercise is to become aware how you are affected by external influences. Begin, perhaps with music. Does a certain genre, or even a specific song, make you feel a certain way? Don't worry about defining exactly how you feel, and certainly don't concern yourself with dissecting why it makes you feel that way. Simply be aware that a certain experience evokes a specific response in you.

Later, when it comes time to adjust negative behaviors, your ability to associate conditions and responses will help you best target those aspects of your external/internal relationship to achieve the behavior and subsequent results that you have established as your goals. If you cannot associate between the external, and your own internal response, then you shall forever remain the hapless victim of your environment.

Start listening to certain music (or eating certain food, visiting certain locations) with the specific intent of altering your state of being in a predictable manner. Harnessing these influences is the first step to decoupling yourself from them, and ultimately towards self mastery.

Meditate: Now, don't let this word distract you. We have gone so insane over this word time and again that it's lost all sense to most people. People say things like "I meditate every day" -or- "I never learned how to meditate". That's like people saying they 'do' yoga; it simply makes no sense. Meditation is any means to arrive at a state of unoccupied consciousness. It may entail breathing exercises, body positions, chanting, mantra, or other sounds. It may invoke a mandala or some other systematic approach...it may also be as simple as watching water drip from a faucet, playing an instrument, or going for an ambling walk. It's not the act of meditation that's important, it's the state of mind one achieves that matters most.

What does that state of mind feel like? Think about those periods just before you fall asleep at night, or that wonderful floating feeling when you become half awake in the morning...it feels a lot like that. Clear, calm, centered. Thoughts can come and go without leaving any distinct impression on your deeper self. Fears are free to make themselves known to your conscious without causing alarm or shame. Hopes and dreams likewise have free expression within your psyche. Your mind is powerful and sharp in this state and is capable of direct action on your body and conscious self.

For most people, meditation isn't so much about 'how to begin', but rather realizing the ways in which you already meditate. Begin to recognize the natural meditative state you employ already in your life (even if it's merely the 'cleansing breath'). By knowing what it feels like when you employ meditation, you will learn to recognize further instances of it in your life, and then eventually to employ those techniques mindfully.

Conclusion

NLP is a system of ordering your experiences, responses, goals, and actions in order to bring them into alignment with your desired results. It is, at its foundation, simply the application of your incredibly powerful self. The techniques focus primarily on focused centered action and clearly defined attainable goals. The tools utilized in achieving these results can easily be trained and improved in your daily life without any special training, they simply require awareness and practice. Because nearly every aspect of your existence stems initially from your own mindset, the ability of NLP to alter your reality i nearly limitless. Illness, doubt, disease, fear, success, greatness, goodness…these are all factors within your realm of control. You can decide which to embrace, which to adjust. You can decide the course of your action, and by directing your action, determine your results. The power is yours, only you must have the courage to wield it.

Thank You Page

I want to personally thank you for reading my book. I hope you found information in this book useful and I would be very grateful if you could leave your honest review about this book. I certainly want to thank you in advance for doing this.

If you have the time, you can check my other books too.

www.ingramcontent.com/pod-product-compliance
Ingram Content Group UK Ltd.
Pitfield, Milton Keynes, MK11 3LW, UK
UKHW021510141125
8981UKWH00039B/448